Everything you need to know about salt

Benefits - Recipes - Body care - Therapies

Anne Pelland

Everything you ever wanted to know about salt! You may not know it or understand it, but as people, we all need a little salt in our lives. From all the way back to the Romans, people have been enjoying salt and the health benefits associated with it.

Who would have thought that something so small and inconsequential is so important to us, if you care about your health and take looking after your body seriously, then it's time that you spent a little bit of time getting back to the basics. Understanding the benefits of salt!

Inside the Benefits of Salt, you'll discover:

- Understanding the Basics of Salt
- The Difference Between Salt & Sea Salt
- Why We Need Salt
- Adding Salt to Your Diet
- Salt Therapy and Salt Treatments
- The Therapeutic Use of Bath Salts
- Natural Salt for Healthy Looking Skin
- How to Use Himalayan Salts for Healing & Much More!

Disclaimer

All Rights Reserved: No part of this publication or the information in it may be quoted from or reproduced in any form by means such as printing, scanning, photocopying or otherwise without prior written permission of the copyright holder.

Disclaimer and Terms of Use: Effort has been made to ensure that the information in this book is accurate and complete, however, the author and the publisher do not warrant the accuracy of the information, text and graphics contained within the book due to the rapidly changing nature of science, research, known and unknown facts, and the internet. The author and publisher assume no liability with respect to losses or damages caused, or alleged to be caused, by any reliance on any information contained herein and disclaim any and all warranties, express or implied, as to the accuracy or reliability of said information.

The publisher and author make no representations or warranties with respect to the accuracy or completeness of the contents of this work and specifically disclaim all warranties. The advice and strategies contained herein may not be suitable for every situation. The Author and the publisher do not hold any responsibility for errors, omissions or contrary interpretation of the subject matter herein. This publication is designed to provide accurate and authoritative information in regard to the subject matter covered and is presented solely for motivational and informational purposes only.

Nothing in this book is a substitute for medical advice nor is it intended to diagnose, treat, cure or prevent any illness or health condition. If you have a condition or health problem, consult your personal health care provider. This book is sold with the understanding that neither the author nor the publisher is engaged in rendering professional services.

Table of Contents

Understanding the Basics of Salt

Believe it or not, salt is essential for life - we literally cannot live without it.

You've heard the saying 'Is he worth his salt?' That saying comes from when the Romans were actually paid in salt! That's where the words 'salary' comes from - 'sal'. We are now paid a 'salary' - all because of salt.

According to Wikipedia, salt is an ionic compound that can be formed by the neutralization reaction of an acid and a base. Salts are composed of related numbers of cations (positively charged ions) and anions (negative ions) so that the product is electrically neutral (without a net charge). These component ions can be inorganic, such as chloride ($Cl-$), or organic, such as acetate ($CH3CO-2$); and can be monatomic, such as fluoride ($F-$), or polyatomic, such as sulfate. The salt potassium dichromate has the bright orange color characteristic of the dichromate anion.

Originally salt was used to kill bacteria that caused food to spoil - therefore it was used as a preservative. Today, however, with refrigeration and other preservatives it is used for other reasons.

Salt also used to be worth its weight in gold - literally! Explorers, both African and European, used to trade an ounce of salt for an ounce of gold. Amazing! So, why then today do we have so much confusion about 'over-salting' our food or the 'high sodium content' in processed food?

Types of Salt

It seems that there are so many different types of salts these days to choose from. You might have thought that salt is just salt, but nothing could be further from the truth! Here is a basic guide to the different types of salt.

Table salt

This is the type of salt that most of us use at home and the type that we find on most restaurant tables. Our basic table salt is made by sending water into salt deposits then evaporating it - only the salt crystals will remain. The salt goes through a refining process that removes the other minerals from it. Table salt has a fine grain texture which makes it ideal for baking - it can accurately be measured.

It contains mostly sodium chloride with additional of iodine. It is currently produced by evaporation of seawater or brine. Usually, it is obtained from brine wells and making use of energy from sunlight. Other than cooking, it is also used in the manufacturing of pulp and paper, produce soap and so on. Recently there are many health issues associated with it, especially high blood pressure.

Kosher

It has a much larger grain size and a more open granular structure. It is coarse-grained and free of additives that tend to cause pickling solutions to the cloud. This type of coarse salt is generally evaporated from brine. This creates grains with a block-structure; this structure better allows the salt crystals to absorb blood (Jewish law states that you must extract blood from meat before you consume it). Kosher salt is less salty than table salt.

Sea salt

It is believed to be better in taste and texture. It is also the coarse and unrefined sea salt that contains many minerals, such as calcium, potassium, magnesium, and sulfate. It generally lacks high concentrations of iodine an element essential for human health; it is not necessarily a healthful substitute for regular iodized table salt

Black salt

It is usually found in Indian markets and sounds uncommon to people in other locations. The characteristic is that it is strong in flavor. The structure is unrefined, and it is actually pinkish gray and has a strong sulfuric flavor. In traditional medicine, it is considered as a cooling spice in Ayurvedic medicine.

Bamboo salt

It is roasted in bamboo and contains more types of minerals balance that is suitable for our body. It is originated from Korean traditional medicine practice. It is believed that it contains the benefit of salt, bamboo and yellow clay that mixed together during the burning process. In order to enhance the benefits, it is repeatedly roasted in bamboo for 3-9 times before it is good for consumption.

Rock salt

It is also called halite and it is inedible. It is the mineral form of Sodium Chloride (NaCl), typically is colorless to yellow, sometime may also in light blue, dark blue, and pink depending on the amount and type of impurities. The primary use is to make ice cream. It is also used to clear highway from icing during winter.

Fleur De Sel

This is a type of sea salt - to harvest fleur de sel, you must take the early crystals that start to form across the surface of salt evaporation ponds - this is generally done during the summer months, the time when the sun is strongest. Fleur de sels have a higher mineral content than basic table salt. Fleur de sels can smell like the ocean, and it tends to be grayish in color. Other types of sea salts include Sel gris, esprit du sel, and pink, black, and brown sea salts from India.

Pickling salt

It is like refined table salt but it does not contain iodine or anti-caking chemicals, both of which turn pickles dark and unsightly. It is virtually 100% sodium chloride. It is a very fine-grained salt and dissolves quickly.

Understanding salt can help us a lot and it is the basic to our health, the reason is simple because everybody needs it. Our body needs it to stay healthy and nutritionally balanced provided we take the correct type. We need more mineral balanced type of salt to maintain the proper function in our body and stay in good health.

The Difference Between Salt Vs Sea Salt

The salt we typically have on our tables and use for cooking has been mined from rock deposits or from Halite, which is the sea salt type.

Nowadays sea salt is harvested from the sea, notably from the Mediterranean, and Atlantic, by the French and Italians. This salt contains minerals including iodine, but table salt has been processed so that it only contains the minerals sodium and chloride. Much of it is then iodized; in other words, the mineral iodine is added to it. Sea salt contains iodine naturally.

Iodizing salt began in the US in the 1920s as an attempt to prevent people from having goiters, an enlargement of the thyroid gland. This has become largely unnecessary as we now know that we can get iodine from dark green vegetables such as spinach, or from algae such as laverbread (also known as the Welshman's caviar). This processed salt has had all minerals removed from it and only contains sodium and chloride, which are the main constituents of all salt.

Sea salt is generally organic and has been harvested by hand, although so is the salt from Pakistan's Khewra mines, the second largest salt mines in the world after Wieliczka in Poland, which is a UNESCO World Heritage Site. A trip to a salt mine is an enlightening experience as the one in Pakistan has buildings, such as a Post Office and a mosque built from bricks of salt. With the lighting effects, the sights to be seen underground are truly remarkable.

In the Indian subcontinent Black salt (Kala namak) is used with fruit such as jamun (Java plums) and falsa (Grewia asiatica), although it is also sometimes used in cooking too. It isn't actually black, but a dirty pink color but I can't eat it as I am put off by the sulfurous smell.

Another salt that comes from Pakistan is Himalayan Crystal salt, which can be found in varying shades of pink. This is one of the 'gourmet' salts, sold for rather exorbitant prices in the rest of the world. It gets its color from the minerals it contains and is said to have the lowest percentage of sodium and chloride of all salts.

The Italian salt, Sale Marino harvested off the coasts of Sicily also contains the minerals magnesium, potassium, and fluorine as well as iodine. French sea salt is also highly thought of and is grey, used on salads, and cooked fresh vegetables as well as grilled meats. Another French salt is Fleur de Sal (Flor de Sal in Portuguese) which comes from the Guérande region of France and is harvested from salt ponds. The weather conditions have to be just right to harvest this salt and it can only be harvested once a year.

Flake salt or Flaky salt is a pretty condiment as it resembles snowflakes a little.

Why we need salt

The main component of salt is sodium. Water and sodium regulate the water content of the body. Both sodium and water are necessary for the proper hydration of our body. We need water inside our cells and also outside our cells. Sodium balances the amount of water that stays outside our cells. Natural salt allows necessary body fluids to freely cross membrane walls (refined salt, however, inhibits this function and can lead to accumulated fluids stagnating in joints and tissues resulting in cellulite, arthritis, rheumatism and kidney problems). Natural salt also balances excess acidity in cells helping to maintain a correct acid/alkaline balance in the body.

Sodium is an electrolyte; a substance that becomes an ion in solution and is able to conduct electricity. Many processes in the brain, nervous system, muscles and other parts of your body use electrical signals for communication. The movement of sodium in your body is essential to the generation of these electrical signals. However, balance is needed, as too much or too little sodium in the body can cause cells to malfunction.

Other common electrolytes include potassium, chloride, and bicarbonate.

The effect of high salt intake

High salt intake is more likely to have a negative effect if you are eating refined table salt. If you eat a diet high in commercial slices of bread and processed foods including flavoring mixes then it is likely that your salt intake is very high. If you eat a diet consisting largely of home prepared foods with a good amount of fresh fruit and vegetables then your salt intake is probably acceptable although you may want to rethink the type of salt that you are using.

High salt (sodium) intake can lead to high blood pressure and increased risk of stroke and heart disease. Excess salt intake (particularly refined salt) can burden the kidneys and adrenal glands, reduce the absorption of nutrients and cause calcium loss. Please note though, that at moderate doses natural salt enhances nutrient and calcium absorption.

Cravings for salt or salty taste can be caused by two main things. Firstly, your salt taste adjusts with consumption. If you eat a lot of salt then it takes higher levels of salt for food to taste salt to you. Secondly, if you eat refined salt, then your body may still crave salt because you are not giving it the absorbable minerals that it needs.

High salt/sodium foods include salted chips and nuts, crackers, bread, baked beans, prepared sauces, prepared flavor mixes, fast foods, prepared meals, anything tinned/bottled in brine (olives, capers, fish) and cheese. Subtle sources of salt and sodium include packaged cakes and biscuits and bottled mineral water.

Who is at risk of not getting enough sodium?

Those at particular risk of having low levels of sodium are people who regularly engage in physically strenuous activities or exercise (ie people who sweat a lot), and those who drink a lot of water and eat little salt. The name for the condition where the body's stores of sodium are too low is called Hyponatremia. The symptoms of Hyponatremia include lethargy, muscle cramps, 'fuzzy' brain and agitation. Confusingly, these symptoms are similar to those of dehydration. If you eat a low salt diet and also consume significant amounts of water, or if you engage in lots of strenuous activity and experience symptoms like these then it is likely that you may need to increase your intake of mineral salt.

Excess saliva (drooling during sleep) may also indicate a deficiency of salt in the body.

Low adrenal function or adrenal exhaustion may also increase your need for salt. Adrenal exhaustion is caused by excessive physical, emotional, environmental and/or psychological stress. "[P]eople with low adrenals have specific problems with their internal water balance... Water poses a specific problem for people with adrenal fatigue because they tend toward dehydration but can easily over dilute the circulating electrolytes (sodium, potassium, magnesium, and chlorine) in their blood by drinking too much water. The balance of sodium and potassium significantly affects the symptoms experienced by people with adrenal fatigue and drinking plain water alters this balance... Therefore, although they are thirsty, drinking water may make them feel worse. To help balance the ratio of water to sodium and avoid this problem try adding 1/4 to 1/2 teaspoon of salt (sodium chloride) to every glass of drinking water. You will probably find that the lightly salted water actually tastes better than regular water if your adrenals are low because the salted water is more beneficial to your body. Certainly, you will feel much better because your body needs both the salt as well as the water. If you are feeling especially draggy or fatigued, add more salt to the water. If you have an aversion to salted water, then you probably need less or no salt in the water"

Quote from Adrenal Fatigue: The 21st Century Stress Syndrome by James L Wilson ND, DC, PhD

Conclusion

Salt is necessary for the proper functioning of our body, but the form of salt is important. Some salts are more easily absorbed and contain higher levels of trace elements than others. Obviously, it is best to go for the most easily absorbed, mineral-rich salt that you can.

In terms of how much salt you need, listen to your body, but generally, it is not much. If you eat a good quality mineral salt then it only takes a small amount to fulfill your body's nutrient needs. A small teaspoon of salt supplies an older child/adult body's daily needs for sodium (infants about 1/4 teaspoon). Sodium is also found in other food ingredients such as sodium bicarbonate (baking soda) and MSG and occurs naturally in many foods.

If possible make most of your food yourself from scratch and then you know the quantity and quality of salt (and sodium) you are ingesting. The best way to consume a balanced amount of salt is to:

- consume largely fresh, raw food (cooked food often uses more salt than raw)

- reduce your meat consumption (meat usually needs a good amount of salt to 'bring out the flavor')

- use lots of natural flavorings like herbs and spices

- avoid fast and pre-prepared food

One thing that salt does is preserve. In other words, salt keeps things from going bad. When Jesus said that we are the salt of the Earth, He was telling us that we are the ones that can keep the world from going completely rotten. We are preserving the work of God on Earth as part of His divine plan to bring restoration and redemption to a dying world.

When we read about the end times when the anti-Christ comes, the only thing that will keep him out of power will be the Spirit-filled believer. As soon as we - the salt - are gone, he takes over. That means, Church, that we need to realize we play a very important part in what happens to this world. God has made us the salt of the Earth.

We take all those buses to the projects because we want to pass the salt in those neighborhoods. We go to Monroe Park because we want to pass the salt to the homeless in Monroe Park. We take the gospel and share the love of Jesus with the prostitutes on the streets of Richmond because Jesus wants us to pass the salt to those forsaken people that He died for on the cross. We go all over the city of Richmond, preaching the gospel because we want to get out of the salt shaker and shake some salt all over our city. Church, if Christians don't do it, it won't happen. The government can't do it. The police department can't do it. Public schools can't save our young people. While it is true that God has salty Christians sprinkled in all of those places, the bottom line is, it is up to Christians to be the salt that is needed to accomplish God's will. It is God's people on assignment throughout the world.

Another quality of salt is that it heals. Before the days of modern medicine and a pill for everything, salt was the cure-all. If you had a cut foot or a splinter in your finger, soaking it in salt water was very healing. Gargling with warm salt water still remains the best thing to do for a sore throat or to promote healing after getting a tooth extracted.

It doesn't take a genius to know that we live in a very sick world. We live in a world that has a spiritual disease and it is getting worse with every passing day. The only cure for the current condition of the world is those who are the salt of the Earth. Don't blame it on Jesus. He said, "Ye are the salt of the Earth." He left us here on a mission to be healing agents to a morally sick and hurting world. It is up to us to pass the salt. Our world is moral, emotionally, spiritually, and physically sick, and we are the salt of the Earth that is so desperately needed. The salt in us is the essence of Christ that abides in us and it is powerful and life-changing.

Salt also adds flavor. One of the main reasons we put salt on our food is because it adds flavor. When you get right down to the truth, the world we live in is very boring. People in the world are bored with the ho-hum of day to day life and are always looking for some action and excitement. Nothing satisfies or adds true flavor to life except Jesus, and it is up to us to make the world taste better. The only way that will happen is if we pass the salt and share Jesus with the lost and forsaken people we encounter in this world. Jesus is the missing ingredient.

Salt doesn't do anything in the shaker. Christians can sit in church every week, but until they take their salt outside the "shaker", they will not do anything for this world. If the only Christianity we live is inside our four walls, we are useless. Jesus had a reason for saying, "GO YE INTO ALL THE WORLD." He knew that's where people are lost, dying, sick, depressed, defeated and living without joy or purpose. It is on us to get outside our four walls and pass the salt... out of our shaker (our comfort zone) and out into the world we live in at work, home, and with those, we meet in our daily walk. Salt is no good until it makes contact with something. We will never be effective out there in a world that is dying and going to Hell until we come into contact with some lost and hurting people and they taste and see the salt in our lives. Get out of your shaker and pass the salt!

Salt loses itself in order to be effective. If salt doesn't lose itself, it would never be effective. Jesus said it in these words in Mark 8:35, "For whosoever will save his life shall lose it; but whosoever shall lose his life for my sake and the gospel's, the same shall save it." He was saying if we really want to effectively be the salt of the Earth, we have to lose whatever is important to us and do that which is important to God. The most important thing to God is that none would perish, and having His children be willing to lay down their lives and generously pass the salt to those He brings into our lives. The only way we can be effective is by losing our will and doing His will.

Salt is no good when it loses its savor. Jesus made it very clear in Matthew 5:13 when He said, "Ye are the salt of the earth: but if the salt has lost his savor, wherewith shall it be salted? It is thenceforth good for nothing, but to be cast out, and to be trodden under foot of men." In other words, we can lose the ability to make a difference. Salt that hasn't lost its savor will make a difference on anything it comes in contact with. Nothing will remain the same once the salt has touched it. It will taste, look, and act differently. That's why Richmond is not the same city it was ten years ago because a lot of people at The ROC decided to start passing the salt around our city. However, when salt loses its savor, it is good for nothing according to Jesus. That is a powerful statement for Jesus to make, but He is right. Savor in the Bible symbolizes the Holy Spirit inside a Christian, which is the power to make a difference. When we lose that saltiness - the power of God in our life - we then become good for nothing when it comes to the work of God. The saddest thing to see is a Christian who has lost the power of God upon their life.

How does that happen? How does salt lose its savor? When rotten elements are mixed with salt, salt loses its savor. When we mix the rotten elements of this world - drugs, alcohol, pornography, lust, greed, gossip, hate, and unforgiveness - it is just a matter of time before our salt will lose its savor.

Salt in Your Diet

Daily recommended Intake = 6g

To keep your body in balance you need a certain amount of salt in your body at any one time. The problem today is most people consume far too much of it. 6g of salt is about a teaspoonful. The average person takes in up to twice this amount each day! 6g is not a large amount when you consider that 75% of the salt we, as a nation, eat comes from everyday processed foods!

When most people think of salt, they think of shaking it on their food or adding a pinch to their cooking. What most of you are unaware of is that processed foods, such as breakfast cereals, soups, biscuits, and ready meals are already loaded with the stuff. Unless you are eating a predominantly clean and healthy diet you are likely to be ingesting a large and unhealthy amount of these crystals on a daily basis.

Excess salt in your diet is likely to raise your blood pressure, because the sodium in salt makes your body retain more water, which creates a greater volume of blood in the blood vessels, leading to a greater build-up of pressure. Your kidneys can also come under attack, as they are designed to remove excess salt from the body, helping to keep our blood pressure normal. Too much salt can gradually damage the kidneys so they become less able to remove this excess sodium.

High blood pressure (hypertension) can be deadly, not least because it often develops with few side effects or symptoms. By the time that it is diagnosed, you may already be at high risk of heart disease or a stroke. Left untreated for too long hypertension can also lead to kidney failure and eye damage.

Eating less salt will lower blood pressure and reduce your risk of heart disease and stroke.

SIMON'S TIPS: SALT

Compare foods and choose low salt content wherever possible. Look at food packaging and see what the salt or sodium content per 100g is. 1.25g or more per 100g (0.5g sodium) indicates a LOT of salt. 0.25g or less per 100g (0.1g sodium or less) indicates a low amount of salt. If a food contains between 0.25g and 1.25g salt (or between 0.1g and 0.5g sodium) per 100g, this is a moderate amount.

Know what foods are generally high in salt: Baked beans, biscuits, breakfast cereals, cooking sauces, hot chocolate, pizza, ready meals, soup, tinned spaghetti, tinned vegetables, anchovies, bacon, cheese, crisps, gravy granules, olives, pickles, pretzels, salted and roasted nuts, sausages, smoked meat and fish, stock cubes, yeast extract (eg: marmite / vegemite).

Aromatherapy Bath Salt

Many believe that the relaxing properties of warm water and well-chosen aromatherapy bath salt can provide relief from unpleasant conditions such as anxiety and stress.

Bath salts are even said has the ability to aid muscle and joint pain, as well as provide relief from the symptoms of many chronic skin conditions.

The best-known aromatherapy bath salts these days is the Dead Sea bath salt. This bath salt is noted as a potent option for seborrhea and psoriasis treatment.

Several studies were conducted to determine the real benefit of this aromatherapy bath salt, and it was discovered that 80 percent of patients affected by psoriasis and osteoarthritis reported less pain after an aromatic bath with the Dead Sea bath salt.

Beside Dead sea salt, there are many salts that use for aromatherapy Bath salts. Such as :

- Sea Salt

- Dendritic Salt

- Epsom salt

- Pickling salt

- European spa salt

- Solar salt

- Breton organic salt

- Hawaiian red salt

- Icelandic brine salt

- Black sea pink salt

Sea Salt

sea salt is simply regular salt with the addition of various minerals present in sea water.Sea salt contain sodium chloride, magnesium and calcium, and other trace elements. The whiter color of sea salt the better. Sea salt is available in fine, medium, and coarse grains. Sea salt is considered a basic salt since it is readily available and generally inexpensive.

Dendritic Salt

Dendritic salt has a unique crystalline form It absorbs and holds the scent in bath salts very efficiently. Dendritic salt is dissolved quickly in your bath water. Without dendritic salt, your bath salt will lose their scent quickly or may form hard lumps. Including a small amount (under 10%) of dendritic salt in each recipe of yours will ensure the scent remains.

Dead Sea Salt

Dead sea salt comes from Israel, is unique in its mineral composition. Much more concentrated than sea salt. Dead sea salt is composed of sodium chloride (like sea salt) plus other mineral and trace elements. Dead sea salt has the ability to totally relax the body and soul just before bedtime. Dead sea salt can be combined with other salts.

Epsom Salt

Epsom salt is a clean and white sparkling salt, Epsom salt color is always the same color from store to store. Epsom is easy to find in your local store. Epsom salt contains magnesium sulfate. It is extracted from bitterns (brine water that has already had sodium chloride removed). So unlike other salts, Epsom salt no contain sodium chloride. Epsom salt is used to ease muscle aches and pain, It is also good for draw toxin from your body.

Pickling salt

Pickling salt is pure and white bright available in medium grain. Easy to find at your local store. Pickling salt is the same as table salt but has three main differences, pickling salt comes in medium grain, so larger than table salt. Pickling salt is not iodized and anti-caking additives. So when you store pickling salt in humid or moist environment, it might form hard lumps.

European spa salt

European spa salt is harvested from the crystal clear waters of the Mediterranean Sea. so it should more expensive than any other salt. European spa salt is evaporated to a sparkling white by the sun and ocean air. European Spas are famous for their in-depth knowledge of natural healing and therapy. It is used for pampering your body in a luxury spa. The composition of this salt is mainly sodium chloride. European spa salt can be mixed with other salts.

Solar salt

Is a white chunky salt. Usually, solar salt is used only as complimentary salt in the recipe because of its size. The large, bright crystal is very attractive if you blend with smaller grain, such as Epsom salt or European spa salt. This salt takes a long time to dissolve in a water. Solar salt is best when blended with other salts.

Hawaiian red salt

Hawaiian Red Salt, also known as Alaea sea salt, is a natural, unprocessed salt. It has a rusty red color because from the red clay present in the area. The volcanic red clay is high in iron oxide. It has curative properties when used for sore throats, wounds, body aches, muscle sprains, gum infections, and cold sores. It is believed to draw toxins from overworked muscle tissue. Hawaiian Red salt can be mixed with other white salts to make the best combination.

Icelandic brine salt

Icelandic Brine Salt comes from a steaming hot (hotter than 300 degrees) pool found 1 mile below the earth's surface in Iceland. This salt is rich in silica and essential trace elements but contains 60% less sodium than regular sea salt. Icelandic Brine Salt dissolves instantly in water and leaves skin feeling silky soft. Use Icelandic Geo-Thermal Brine Salts in your bath to relax sore, tired muscles, detoxify your skin and to help relieve dry, scaling skin conditions. Gentle enough to use in baby's bath water for relieving itchy skin. Use this mineral-rich salt in your creams and lotions for various dry skin conditions. Icelandic Brine Salt can be mixed with other salts.

Black sea pink salt

This salt is harvesting from traditional method to ensure that the salt retains its natural mineral and remains chemical free. High concentrations of halophilic bacteria live in the water and salt crust and cause the pink coloration of this salt.

Black Sea Pink Salt has been said to provide pain relief from eczema, psoriasis, rheumatism, arthritis and muscle strain. It has also been used by the ancients to improve the health of the skin.

Black Sea Pink Salt is a unique luxury salt to use in your bath recipes. You can mix this salt with another salt to make a great combination.

You can make aromatherapy bath salt for yourself or give it to your friends. Aromatherapy bath salt would be the perfect gift for any occasion. With a nice packaging, you will surprise how they react!

Salt Therapy

Salt therapy was discovered in the mid-18th century by Polish health official named Felix Botchkowski. Salt therapy was originally discovered as Speleotherapy or cave therapy, 'Spelenos' being the Greek term for 'cave'. Felix Botchkowski found that salt miners in Poland had not experienced lung-related ailments such as asthma, pneumonia, or chronic bronchitis. Even miners who had the respiratory disease before they began working in the mines felt better and had fewer symptoms as they spent more and more time in the caves. Felix Botchkowski published a book in 1843 on his findings. His predecessor Mstislav Poljokowski founded the first Salt Spa in Velicko, which is still in operation today.

The benefits of salt were also noticed in the 1940's, around the end of World War II. Abandoned salt mines were frequently used as bomb shelters. Those who sought safety in these mines found a reduction in respiratory symptoms. Soon after, salt sanatoriums opened in European countries such as Germany, Hungary, and Yugoslavia. In 1968 the Hospital of Allergic Diseases officially authorized the scientific foundation of Speleotherapy.

Speleotherapy is the treatment of respiratory diseases, as well as some skin diseases, utilizing salt-rich air in underground caves. Natural salt microns and ions have been proven effective in calming an agitated respiratory track. Salt has a natural anti-inflammatory effect; it reduces swelling and edema in the air passages, making it less difficult and less painful to breathe. Inhaling the salt-saturated air destroys fungus and bacteria in the mucosal lining of the respiratory tract. Breathing the salted air thins the mucus in the lungs so it is more easily expectorated. It has also been proven to remove remaining tar from the lungs of smokers. The salt ions produce a negative electrical charge in the air, which improve mood, reduce stress and anxiety, decrease fatigue, and have many other curative effects.

During a treatment, the patient is allowed to relax in the salt cave for the duration of the session. Each session lasts from twenty to forty-five minutes and is repeated daily for up to fifteen days. Treatments are recommended up to three times per year. Speleotherapy treatments are typically not private; patients usually can share a treatment cave with as many as thirty other individuals.

Outside the caves, salt therapy is called Halotherapy. It comes from the Greek word 'halos', a term meaning 'salt'. Halotherapy is essentially a replication of Speleotherapy, using a dry aerosol spray to coat the walls and ceiling of a room. Man-made salt rooms allow the opportunity for a private session, but larger salt room is built to accommodate many more patients.

Halotherapy can also be used privately at home. A device called a salt pipe, a personal dry-salt inhaler, can be used daily for up to twenty-five minutes. An air salitizer is another way to gain the same benefits of salt therapy. They negatively charge the room in the same manner as a salt mine. "The Salin device is a bionic air purifier, natural ionizer and salinizer that uses forced ionization of the indoor air by salt sublimation (places tiny microparticles of salt into the air). The salt microcrystals are under 5µm diameter, with a majority under 1µm and are able to penetrate deep into the lung." Salt lamps are also an easy way to change the electric charge in the room. The heat from the light bulb or candle inside the lamp sends off the negatively charged salt ions. This cleans the air in the room. The salt ions cling to airborne allergens making them heavy, allowing them to fall out of the air so they don't get breathed in. The negative ions improve mood and reduce stress and anxiety.

Speleotherapy and Halotherapy have been effective in reducing symptoms in many areas of health. Although treatments are most used to remedy lung-related disorders, salt has also been used to care for skin conditions, anxiety, stress, ENT illnesses, and has been utilized to improve the immune system. Conditions that are treated with salt include, but are not limited to:

• Asthma

• Allergic colds, Hay Fever, and Rhinopathy

• Chronic bronchitis

• Sinusitis

• Frequent viral infections

• Frequent ear infections

• Chronic Obstructive Pulmonary Disease

• Smoker's cough

• Tonsillitis

• Snoring

• Psoriasis

• Eczema

• Stress and anxiety disorders

• Insomnia

• Arthritis

• Cystic Fibrosis

Salt therapy falls under the class of physical therapies. It is a non-invasive, natural therapy without the side effects of drugs normally used to treat these ailments, such as corticoids or steroids. The absence of these drugs allows this treatment to be safe for pregnant women, and even very young children. Children that receive this therapy inhale a lower concentration of salt air.

The Holistic Method Of Salt Therapy For Asthma

Often when people hear the word "salt", images of high blood pressure and heart disease come to mind but really, good health is dependent upon the proper balance of natural salts. Therefore, adopting the natural holistic method of salt therapy is essential to maintaining a resistance to free radicals and toxins within the body.

Iodized table salt from the grocery store not taken in moderation can have detrimental effects on the body. It thickens the blood which in turn makes the heart pump harder to push the blood through the arteries and capillaries. This is one of the root causes of heart disease. However, natural crystalline sea salt has many powerful antioxidants and can stave off the effects and help to normalize blood pressure, whether it is high or low. A good salt therapy is also used as an alternative asthma therapy due to the fact that sea salt is a natural antihistamine.

Placing natural salt on the tongue and consuming a few glasses of water helps to reduce the effects of asthma and provides relief from dry hacking coughs. Typically, hacking coughs come as the result of phlegm in the throat and the thicker it is, the longer the cough will last; the salt thins the mucus and stops the cough. There are so many advantages to adopting a good salt therapy regimen. Because our bodies are made up of mostly salt and water, replenishing them often will help reduce the effects of osteoporosis and Alzheimer's Disease in addition to being a good alternative asthma therapy.

How exactly does salt therapy treat asthma?

The patient will be placed in a comfortable chair in a special room for one hour. Here is where the salt therapy will be conducted.

Each hour constitutes one session and the patient will be asked to breathe normally while listening to relaxing music. As the person breathes in the air in the room, tiny salt particles which are negatively ionized will enter the respiratory system reaching even the deepest portions of the lungs.

As the dry saline aerosol is inhaled during salt therapy, inflammation of the respiratory tract is reduced. Edema, found in the mucosa of the airway passages, is absorbed and this leads to a widening of these passages. When this occurs, mucus will be transported normally again and anything blocking the passage will become unclogged. This helps to remove any foreign allergens and residual tar from the bronchi and bronchioles.

As the respiratory system clears itself, patients using salt therapy can breathe easier. This benefits the patient in many ways. Not only will the quality of life be improved, but fewer medications will also be needed. Hospitalizations will be less likely to happen and the number of asthma attacks will decrease. This treatment option can be used by those of any age.

Salt therapy has been shown to be very effective when used properly. Over 57% of those who have tried this treatment method say that they are able to cut back on their use of prescription medications. Eighty percent suffer less dyspnoea and it is shown to be up to 98% effective. Benefits of this treatment method may last up to 12 months or longer and fewer sick days are needed, an average of 11 fewer. This is one treatment that anyone suffering from asthma should try to see how it can benefit you.

There are so many wonderful advantages to adopting the holistic approach of salt therapy. Taken in moderation, it is very good for you and can help reduce the effects of high blood pressure and heart disease. Doctors with good holistic therapy acumen also tout the benefits of salt in regulating emotional disorders such as depression. It is important to note, though, that those with existing kidney and heart conditions should speak with their doctors before adopting any type of holistic approach. While these methods can be very advantageous, they can also be detrimental to those with medically treated conditions so it would be very astute of the patient to notify their doctor when considering this approach.

Cystic Fibrosis and The Salt Therapy Benefits

Cystic fibrosis is a disease which affects most secretory glands such mucus and sweat glands. The organs and parts of the body most affected include the lungs, liver, sinuses, pancreas and the exocrine glands.

CF is a genetic illness that occurs because of the mutation within the CFer gene on chromosome 7.

When having this illness, the mucus becomes thick and very sticky and this interferes with the normal functioning and clearance of the mucus. This allows for bacteria to grow which leads to various infections that can take place within the lungs, pancreas and sinus cavities.

Cystic Fibrosis Symptoms

They may vary from person to person, where some symptoms may be bad on one day and then eased up on the next day.

Sufferers have very thick mucus build-ups within the airways, which is the perfect breeding ground for bacteria causing infections. Lung infections are very common for cystic fibrosis sufferers, whereby if left untreated it may lead to severe liver damage. Patients may also suffer from repeated bouts of sinus infection, bronchitis, and even pneumonia.

Over time, the illness may lead to pancreatitis, rectal prolapse, gallstones, and even diabetes.

Other signs of cystic fibrosis include infertility, abnormal salty sweat, low bone density and a complete imbalance of minerals within the body.

Cystic Fibrosis Treatment

With no complete cure available at this point in time, CF treatments include:

• Chest physical therapy.

• Working with a team of specialists including dieticians, social workers, and medical specialists to determine personal treatments options.

• Use of medications such as antibiotics, anti-inflammatories, and mucus-thinning medications.

Cystic Fibrosis and Salt Therapy

As patients with cystic fibrosis struggle to breathe, suffer from lung infections, coughing, chronic sinus infection, advances in research has allowed sufferers to utilize hypertonic saline treatments in easing symptoms.

A study held in Australia concluded that CF sufferers who surfed (and they were essentially exposed to the sea-shore salt aerosol) suffered less lung infections and breathing issues than those who didn't. Another study on the effects of hypertonic saline aerosol on cystic fibrosis patients stated that "Hypertonic saline treatment is associated with an improvement in lung function and marked benefits with respect to exacerbations. It appears broadly applicable as an inexpensive therapy for most patients with CF."

Salt Therapy - Effective Alternative Way To Cure Bronchitis

Nowadays, the cost of being sick is very expensive between the cost of seeing the doctor, getting the necessary x-rays or treatment and the cost of medicine if needed. Not only is it costly but very annoying. If by chance you have a disease that requires ongoing treatment, it can rack up into the $1,000s. For those with no insurance and a bad illness, it's never a good scenario.

Governments do help by offering health plans for the needy like children and older adults. You can find these programs by going to your local organizations that do offer free health care services.

After so tries at many medications, people tend to resort to natural remedies. Also, many people gravitate towards this resort because of the effects of the medicine.

One such therapy people try is Halotherapy or what is initially called to salt therapy or speleotherapy. Overseas in Europe, this is a well-documented type of therapy. This was well practiced in the early 19th century in the salt mines. Today, physicians are trying to duplicate its effect by using dry aerosol salt particles and minerals.

It was recognized by Felix Botchkowi, a health official, that salt miners never got lung-related diseases. During World War II, salt mines were turned into shelters and those who had asthma tended to feel much better. There are still salt hospitals in various parts of the world including Russia, Poland, Romania, and Austria

The best thing about salt-therapy is it's non-invasive and no drug therapy of the respiratory diseases. That does include bronchitis. While medicine therapy does have its advantages and disadvantages, salt therapy is a natural means with no side effects. Clinical trials are being tested worldwide for the salt therapy benefits.

Respiratory diseases are a major cause of morbidity globe wide. Most drug therapies have slight side effects while steroid treatments have greater ones. No doubt with the side effects, that salt therapy is a great "natural" possible cure. No wonder there is a need for salt.

Diabetes Treatment With Cupping And Pure Salt Therapy

There are two types of diabetes namely diabetes insipidus and diabetes mellitus.

Diabetes insipidus is a rare metabolic disorder in which the patient produces large quantities of urine and is constantly thirsty. It is due to a deficiency of the pituitary hormone vasopressin, an antidiuretic hormone which regulates reabsorption of water in the kidneys. Treatment is by administration of vasopressin to the patient and cannot be treated by Cupping and Pure Salt therapy as the pituitary glands are located deep inside the brain.

Diabetes mellitus affects about 7% of the general population and can be divided into type 1 (insulin-dependent) and type 2 (non-insulin-dependent). Type 1 accounts for about 10% while type 2 represent 90 % of all diabetes mellitus. Type 1 normally affect children and teenagers which have little or no ability to produce the hormone insulin and patients are entirely dependent on insulin injections for survival. The hormone insulin is produced by the pancreas and helps to regulate the blood sugar level when it exceeds the preset limit. It is thought that type 1 is caused by damage to the pancreas tissues that produce insulin due to misplaced attack of the pancreas by the patient's own immune system (autoimmune attack). Cupping and Shin Gum Pure Salt therapy cannot treat type 1 because of permanent damage to the pancreas.

Type 2 being the most common diabetes was prevalent amongst patients in the middle and old age. However, in recent years the number of young people suffering from type 2 diabetes has increased. It can be found in young people in the twenties and thirties. Type 2 diabetes is due to inadequate production of insulin to meet the needs of the patient or the result of the body becoming resistant to the effects of insulin. The accumulation of sugar leads to its appearance the blood (hyperglycemia) and then in the urine. Symptoms include thirst, excessive production of urine, aging and itching skin, loss of sensation, loss of teeth, blurring of vision, constant hunger, and loss of weight due to the use of body fats as an alternative source of energy to sugar. Risk factors include incidence in family members (genetics), obesity, lack of exercise, sedentary lifestyle, diabetes during pregnancy and unhealthy eating habits (too much sugar, excessive carbohydrates, overeating).

Long-term complications of type 2 diabetes include higher risk of heart attack (myocardial infarction) and stroke attack (cerebrovascular accident), highest incidence of blindness due to damage of blood vessels supplying the optic nerve (diabetic retinopathy), highest cause of kidney failure requiring dialysis (diabetic nephropathy), thigh pain and progressive weakness of knee extension (diabetic amyotrophy), pain or numbness of the feet due to nerve damage (diabetic neuropathy), amputation of legs due to gangrene, and impotence due to damage nerves of the penis (erectile dysfunction).

Type 2 diabetes can be treated with cupping of points 2, 3, 6 and 8 with only 30% success rate due to the fact that the pancreas is located deep inside the viscera behind the liver. However, a much higher success rate is achieved by applying Aggressive Cupping combine with Pure Salt therapy. For diabetes type 2 Pure Salt therapy comprise of daily one hour exercise, gradual reduction of food followed by fasting, daily pure salt half-body bath, consumption of pure salt (preferably 200-hour pure salt or minimum 30-hr pure salt), stress reduction techniques and adopting a positive mental attitude to diabetes.

Homeopathic Treatments - Effective Salt and Saline Treatments for Cold and Flu Symptoms

A non-pharmacological therapy for sinus congestion and sinus infections, as well as allergic rhinitis, is nasal saline irrigation, a treatment which has been known for centuries to be effective in preventing and treating these conditions. The American Academy of Allergy Asthma and Immunology suggests saline sinus rinse as a treatment for chronic or acute sinus infections and allergic rhinitis, stating that irrigation of sinus cavities with salt can "bring relief by removing allergens from the nostrils and sinuses". They also suggest using salts that contain no iodide, anti-caking agents or preservatives which can irritate the nasal lining. Some of the salts you can use to avoid these irritants are Pickling Salts or Himalayan Sea Salts, the latter being readily and conveniently available together with a device called a Neti Pot for this specific use.

Salt Air Therapy is the process of breathing air containing dry, micronized salt particles which travel to all areas of the lungs providing a natural way to cleanse and maintain the respiratory system from within. This all natural, safe and effective therapy helps to reduce inflammation in the airways effectively reducing constriction in the sinuses and lungs that can occur with colds and flus, as well as asthma, allergies and other sinus conditions. By helping the body to naturally eliminate allergens and pollutants, Salt Air Therapy also helps to support the body's immune system. This treatment is most effective when large quantities of time are spent inhaling dry salt air. Due to its rather unique ability to be procured in large chunks, which can be fashioned into blocks or used in natural crystal form, Himalayan Salt is largely prevalent in

Salt Air Therapy. Himalayan Salt Caves have been constructed at many locations worldwide, including several in the US, for Salt Air Therapy. Patrons of these caves spend anywhere between 45 minutes to several hours in the caves in order to breath the salt air. However, it is usually not practical, or even possible, for individuals to travel to a salt cave on a regular basis, let alone stay for large quantities of time. The most convenient and available method of salt air therapy is the Salt Air Inhaler, which is also readily found online and in stores accompanied by Himalayan Sea Salt. Himalayan Salt lamps, chunks of salt which have been made into lamps by installing a bulb inside of a hole drilled into the bottom of a salt crystal and mounted onto a wooden base, can also be placed around the home for increased exposure to ionized salt air.

Gargling with a salt water solution has been known to reduce swelling and irritation associated with a sore or irritated throat and cough since antiquity. This natural treatment helps to reduce harmful bacteria, thereby treating and preventing infection with anti-bacterial and anti-microbial properties. Himalayan Salt Glasses provide a convenient method for preparing salt water solution for gargling, by simply filling the glass with water and allowing a few moments for some of the salt to dissolve into the water. This method provides a natural, pure salt solution for gargling with unprocessed salts which do not possess added iodide, caking agents or preservatives.

Proper irrigation of the ear canal with a saline solution helps to cleanse the canal of wax and treat and/or minimize the risk of bacterial infection. This is best performed by mixing three parts of water with one part salt, then administering the solution to the ear canal via a bulb syringe. Again, salt which does not contain caking agents or preservatives should be used for this homeopathic treatment. Q-tips should not be used to clear wax from the ear canal due to potential damage to the eardrum; cleaning the ear canal with Q-tips can also push wax further into the ear.

Most of these simple Homeopathic, Holistic and Natural salt treatments have been noted by many cultures since antiquity for their ability to effectively treat ailments and even prevent health issues from arising. Since these methods have been tried and tested throughout the ages for effectiveness, they are an excellent choice for those dealing with the symptoms of colds and flus, as well as the other ailments mentioned. Unlike other traditional treatments, these require no special knowledge of preparation or usage, allowing the use of these remedies by anyone who wishes to enjoy their benefits

Bath Salts' Therapeutic Use

Sea salt and seawater have been proven as the basis of many kinds of therapeutic treatments. There are many kinds of Water Therapy treatment. These include spas, ayurvedic & holistic centers, and health clinics all over the world. Some sports therapy clinics prefer to use Hydrotherapy Baths to help their patients recover from various muscle and joint injuries. Dermatologists also recommend the use of Dead Sea Salt baths for patients with such diseases like Psoriasis, eczema and other skin diseases or problems.

Estheticians emphasize that the cleansing properties of a sea salt bath include cleaning pores and detoxification of the body as well. Many patients with cancer are advised by doctors to use water therapy. They should also use water therapies to help them deal with radiation treatments. There are many kinds of water therapies & therapeutic bath salts that you can use every day or every week in your own house.

The Father of Medicine, Hippocrates, discovered the therapeutic qualities of Sea Water. He noticed the healing effects of it when a fisherman was injured and the sea salt helped treat his wounds. The Sea Water is not only for treating skin diseases or curing an infection, but it is also a great stress reliever. Patients who used these treatments have experienced pain relief and stress relief. That is why it has been now proven that sea salt therapy is a very effective treatment that assists the cells in rejuvenating and can also remove toxins from the body and induces minerals to the body.

Natural Salt For Healthy Skin

Did you know you can use salt to give your skin a healthy glow? Salt is an ancient, natural beauty secret! But don't reach for the refined sodium chloride table salt in your salt shaker. You'll need Original Himalayan Crystal Salt, which still retains its full spectrum of beneficial minerals.

The most effective natural salt for skin treatments is that mined in the majestic Himalayan Mountains. Millions of years ago - when our planet Earth was a pristine ecosystem - a primordial sea was evaporated by the sun, leaving absolutely pure crystalline salt that contains the 84 minerals and trace elements essential to health. Today, this salt still retains the bioenergetic qualities of an unpolluted planet.

Here's how natural salt works to beautify your skin. Skin protects the internal functions of our bodies from outside influences and is our body's largest organ of purification. To function optimally, our skin needs neutral pH factors. Most skin care products from the cosmetics industry make our skin more acid. Natural salt can regulate the pH of the skin to its optimum level through its balancing and neutralizing effects.

HEALING PROBLEM SKIN

Acne, unhealthy skin, and eczema can all be greatly helped by the application of salt mixed with water. This releases the healing properties of natural salt.

To make the salt solution, add enough original Himalayan crystal salt stones to pure water to fully saturate the water with salt. You can tell when the water is fully saturated because you cannot dissolve any more salt into the water, and the salt crystals will just sit in the bottom of the glass. Use a coarse ground salt or salt stones. Place them in the bottom of a glass, add water, and allow the salt to dissolve. If it dissolves completely, add more. When the salt crystals will no longer dissolve, the water is fully saturated. An 8-ounce glass of water will take several tablespoons of salt.

Once a day apply this salt solution to the troubled areas and allow it to absorb into the skin. Do not use any creams or other skin treatments.

Twice a week, mix this salt solution with powdered clay to make a mud mask. Apply the mask to your skin and let it soak in for 15-20 minutes, then remove the dried mask with a wet washcloth.

Though initial worsening of the skin is possible, once this phase passes, the skin improves dramatically.

BATHING BEAUTY

Though many "bath salts" made of refined salt and artificial fragrances are sold, natural salt in the bath has real beauty and health benefits.

Unlike regular baths, which pull moisture from the skin, the upper callous layer of the skin absorbs and holds salt from the natural salt bath, binding water and bringing moisture into the skin. This maintains the skin's natural protective film and keeps the skin from drying out.

In addition, toxins from the body are released into the bath water through osmosis, while the minerals from the salt are absorbed through the skin. A 30-minute bath containing natural salt has the detoxifying effects of a three-day fast!

To make a natural salt bath, you'll need two pounds of the original Himalayan crystal salt for an average-size bathtub. Pour the entire contents of the bag into your bathtub. Add enough water to just cover the salt and let it dissolve for a half hour. Then fill your bathtub with body temperature water (98.6 degrees - check it with a thermometer). Do not add any other bath products - just the salt. Soak 15-30 minutes.

If you want to optimize the benefits of the original Himalayan crystal salt bath, take a bath to absorb minerals at the new moon and a bath to detox the body at the full moon.

Bath Salts for Rejuvenating Instantly

Bath salts are crystalline granules good for rejuvenating bodies instantly. Providing warm therapeutic experiences they drain away the tension and stress of your body to have you in good condition. Designed to clean and refurbish tired bodies, these cosmetic agents are also curative in nature. Aside from enhancing bathing experiences they provide medicinal benefits.

You now get salts that mimic properties of natural mineral baths or hot springs. The addition of fragrances and colors makes them act as diluents to also offer soothing aromas. Other additives include oils that come in the form of bath oil beads and may also be foaming or effervescent agents. Almost everybody loves using them to help get relaxed while taking nice hot baths.

Decidedly they make you feel rejuvenated anytime - winters or summers. You can indulge in lovely aromatherapy baths by soaking in salts providing pure pleasure. With exciting recipes for making all kinds of home concoctions, you actually save money even as you provide yourself special treats. Simply combine different ingredients to create unique blends as per your personal choice. That is the benefit of making them yourself.

It is possible that you will be able to find basic salts in a bulk bin in grocery stores but you may have a hard time finding the necessary oils and fragrances needed for your bath salts recipes. So then it does make sense buying them straight off the shelf. Also, keep them dry before use to stop them from going hard.

For those of us who are stressed for a time it's the stores or pharmacies that will offer relaxing bath salts to help relieve sore muscles and ease tension with an assortment of ready-made packaged stuff. Buy them easily online. A word of caution though, never buy it in bulk as they have a history of clumping and losing scents.

Also remember special salts or aromatherapy ingredients using perfumes and scented oils will in time, under certain conditions have the scents fading away. It is useful to store them in glass containers and not in paper or plastic boxes. It is also recommended to store them in a cool, dry place out of direct sunlight.

Epsom salts are well known for relieving sore muscles. The magnesium sulfate content fights lactic acid in muscles providing relaxation and relief from all the soreness. It is suggested that you do not shower after using Epsom bath salts so the skin can benefit even after you finish bathing. Also, do not use any other product when using Epsom bath salts.

You can make use of them any time you have a bath but using them for night time baths will help you relax and unwind and would certainly be the best time. For a relaxing and sedative bath, you can soak two cups of Epsom salt in warm water. Also massage handfuls of Epsom Salt over your wet skin, from feet up to your face to rinse off and feel wonderful.

Natural Sea Salts a Key to Rejuvenation

Your body is 75% water... and this water that is in your very blood, tissues, and cells contain salts. People may have blamed it for many sicknesses of the body, but salt is an essential part of life itself that flows in your very body.

Salt Wars: Table Salts or Sea Salts?

Salts are made when sea water is exposed to the sun. The table salts we use today are mostly refined, which is stripped off a variety of healthy minerals found on the unrefined ones. During the kiln-drying process, good minerals such as calcium, potassium, and magnesium are removed at high heat. This process makes the salt hard on the body which leads to high blood pressure, heart problems, kidney diseases and many more.

Restore the Body's Balance with Natural Sea Salts?

Going natural will surely give you a lot of healthful benefits, such as:

A Stabilized Blood Pressure

Removal of excess acid from the body's cells

A balanced Blood Sugar Level

Better absorption of food

Energy for the body

Clear Lungs and Ease in Breathing

Prevention of Muscle Cramps

Sea Salts for breathing discomforts? Your folks may have been right to let you sniff a cup of hot water with a dash of salt on those days when you can't breathe from nasal congestion, allergic rhinitis, and some minor lung disease. Halotherapy or Salt Therapy had been popularly used in Eastern Europe. This therapy involves breathing salt air, believed to be good for the lungs.

Sea Salts for bathing? Sea Salts are used in bath therapy to alleviate skin infections and enhance cell rejuvenation. It is even applied on the body for massage. Researchers have noticed an improvement on one's immune system after a natural sea salt bath therapy.

How to Use Himalayan Salt for Healing

Himalayan salt has long been used by many people to alleviate symptoms of different health conditions even before modern medicines were formulated. It provides an all-natural remedy from skin diseases to menstrual cramps to respiratory problems. This salt is commonly used in a solution form, or a brine, which is basically the mixture of the salt crystals and water. This brine solution provides a detoxifying effect on the body. When used topically, as a bath soak, for example, it can help stimulate natural cell growth in your cell layers. As an effect, your body will feel more balanced and your energy flow will be activated. While anyone can benefit from a Himalayan brine bath, it is particularly beneficial to those with various skin diseases, gynecological conditions, rheumatism, and recurring infections.

To get the full benefits of a healing Himalayan salt bath, you have to find the right balance between the water and the salt. The salt concentration has to be at least the same as your body fluids, which is approximately 1 percent, to successfully activate the osmotic exchange ratio. A regular bathtub normally takes from 100 liters of water so in that case, you'll need about a kilo of Himalayan salt to get the right salt concentration. However, if you don't have a bathtub or if you don't have that much natural salt available at home, then don't fret. There are other ways to use Himalayan salt aside from soaking your whole body in it. Let me share to you other ways on how you can use Himalayan salt for healing.

1. Body Scrub. To do this, mix about three tablespoons of Himalayan salt with a tablespoon of natural oil such as virgin coconut oil or olive oil. Take a warm shower first to open up your

pores and then apply the salt scrub to your body. Not only does this improve your circulation, but it also purifies your skin. People with skin asthma, psoriasis, and other skin conditions can greatly benefit from this. While scrubbing your skin, you may experience a warm flow throughout your body. This only shows that your body cells have begun their work. Rinse it all off with lukewarm water after.

2. Himalayan salt is an excellent product for dental hygiene. It can help maintain the right PH balance in your mouth which can help prevent bad breath, gum disease, and tooth decay. To use it, brush your teeth every morning using a Himalayan salt brine. Gargle for about three minutes then spit it out.

3. Drinking good quality water mixed with a teaspoon of Himalayan brine can also help treat various health conditions such as Psoriasis and Herpes, just to name a few. Taking it internally is an excellent way to detoxify and activate your metabolism. If you're scared of the idea of drinking salt, don't be. First of all, it's not like your regular table salt, it is a natural salt. Besides, it's been diluted twice so you can really barely taste its saltiness.

Salt Recipes

Sprouts Curry - A Delicious Low Salt Recipe for Hypertension Patients!

High Blood Pressure Low Salt Recipes

SPROUTS KADHI

Preparation time 15 minutes

Cooking time 15 minutes

Serves 4

INGREDIENTS

1 cup mixed sprouts (moong, chana, makai), cooked

1/2 tsp cumin seeds (jeera)

1/4 tsp mustard seeds (rai/sarson)

2 bay leaves (tejpatta)

2 whole red chilies broken into pieces

1/8 tsp asafetida (hing)

1 tsp ginger-green chili paste

½ tsp red chili powder

¼ tsp turmeric powder (haldi)

2 cups low-fat curds (dahi)

4 tsp besan (Bengal gram flour)

2 tsp oil

¼ tsp salt

Let's check out the recipe for Sprouts Curry, a low salt dish for hypertension patients.

For this, we need precooked mixed sprouts.

FOR THE KADHI (CURRY), we need curd which is nicely stirred.

FOR THE TEMPERING, we need bay leaves, dry red chilies, and mustard seeds.

We need salt to taste, a teaspoon of coarsely grounded ginger and chili.

We also need two pinches of asafetida and a little gram flour.

People often make 'Kadhi'.

There is 'Sindhi Kadhi' and 'Maharashtrian Kadhi'. In UP there are some different Kadhis.

But this particular Kadhi is meant especially for high blood pressure patients and uses sprouts very smartly. There are all sprouts in it.

First, we will mix the gram flour and curd. Mix it nicely such that there are no lumps.

Add in a bit of water.

While adding water, keep in mind that you do not need to add a lot of water. Just add a little water and bring the mixture to a lumpy formation.

Then you can add some more water so as to prevent lumpy formation.

We are done.

TEMPERING:

Now we will heat some oil in a pan.

Add in some mustard seeds for the tempering.

We will add coarsely grounded green chilies and ginger paste once the mustard seeds start crackling.

Now add in bay leaves, red chilies and a bit of asafetida.

Asafetida has its distinct flavor but you have to be a little careful while adding it.

Asafetida will burn if you suddenly put it in the oil.

So we put all other ingredients and then add asafetida. That way, it won't get burnt and you will find its taste as well.

Now we will add the mixture of curd and gram flour into the pan.

Add in some water to monitor the thickness of the mixture.

Upon cooking for some time, you can add in the sprouts.

Lots of sprouts! Wow!

Now let's add in salt.

Add salt at the very end because we are using curd, green gram and after that, we had added dry spices.

Then we added in the sprouts.

If we add salt to the curd, then it would've been insufficient for the sprouts.

That's why we add all the ingredients and then add salt to taste.

You must keep in mind that this is a low salt recipe and a recipe which is being made for the people with high blood pressure. So you must use salt in a limited quantity.

Our 'Sprouted Kadhi' is ready.

Now we will serve it. It looks amazing.

When you serve, choose to keep the bay leaf and red chili towards the top.

Salt Roasted Summer Vegetables

What you need:

- 2 red apples, peeled, seeded and sliced into 8 pieces

- 4 cups unpeeled gold potatoes, cut into 1 1/2-inch piece

- 2 cups peeled carrots, cut into 1 1/2-inch piece

- 2 cups peeled butternut squash, cut into 1 1/2-inch piece

- 2 cups peeled red sweet potatoes, cut into 1 1/2-inch piece

- 2 cups peeled white sweet potatoes, cut into 1 1/2-inch piece

- 2 cups red onion, cut into 1 1/2-inch wedge

- 16 2-inch fresh thyme sprigs

- 8 fresh flat leaf parsley sprigs, coarsely torn

- 1/2 cup olive oil

- 1 teaspoon fine sea salt, divided

- 1 teaspoon crushed red pepper flakes

Soak potatoes, butternut squash, red potatoes, and white potatoes in separate containers for 10-15 minutes then drain. Place the vegetables in a large bowl and add the olive oil. Toss to coat. Add 3/4 teaspoon of the sea salt, red pepper flakes, and thyme sprigs. Spread the vegetables in a 12x18 inch rimmed sheet pan and bake in a pre-heated oven (400 degrees F) for 25 to 30 minutes. Add apples, stir and bake for 30 minutes more or until apples and vegetables are brown and tender. Transfer to serving bowl, top with remaining sea salt and garnish with parsley.

Butter and Sea Salt Grilled Sea Bass

What you need:

- 1 kg. sea bass

- 2 cloves garlic, chopped

- 3 tablespoons butter

- 1 1/2 tablespoons extra virgin olive oil

- 1 tablespoon chopped Italian flat leaf parsley

- 1/4 teaspoon sea salt

- 1/4 teaspoon garlic powder

- 1/4 teaspoon onion powder

- Lemon pepper to taste

- Paprika to taste

Melt the butter in a small saucepan over medium heat and cook garlic and parsley for about 30 seconds. Remove from heat and set aside. Combine sea salt, garlic powder, onion powder, lemon pepper and paprika in a small bowl. Rub the mixture onto the fish. Place the sea bass in heavy duty aluminum foil then grill over high heat for 5 to 7 minutes. Turn, drizzle with butter then cook for 5 to 7 minutes more or until fish is easily flaked with a fork. Drizzle with olive oil then serve.

Sea Salt and Parmesan Asparagus

What you need:

- 1/2 kg. asparagus spears, trimmed and cut into 1 1/2-inch piece

- 1 lemon, juiced and zested

- 1/2 cup shredded Parmesan cheese

- 3 tablespoons butter, melted

- 1 teaspoon minced garlic

- 3/4 teaspoon ground black pepper

- 1/2 teaspoon sea salt

Place asparagus in a medium bowl then add lemon juice and zest, Parmesan, butter, garlic, black pepper, and sea salt. Toss to coat evenly. Arrange spears in a baking dish evenly. Bake in a pre-heated oven (400 degrees F), stirring occasionally, for 10 to 15 minutes or until asparagus spears are tender.

POHA HANDWA

Preparation Time 30 minutes

Cooking Time 20 minutes

Makes 4 Handwas

INGREDIENTS

1 cup jada poha (thick beaten rice flakes)

1/2 cup low fat curds with 1 1/2 cups water

1/2 cup grated white pumpkin (doodhi/lauki)

1/2 cup grated carrots

1/4 cup boiled green peas

1 tbsp green chili-ginger paste

1 tsp sugar

2 pinch turmeric powder (haldi)

2 pinch red chili powder

FOR THE TEMPERING

1 tsp mustard seeds (rai/sarson)

2 tsp sesame seeds (til)

2 pinch asafoetida (hing)

1 tsp oil

OTHER INGREDIENTS

2 tsp oil for cooking

1/4 tsp salt

You might know what Handwa is. You might've had a Handwa sometime.

But handwa made of beaten rice! It's different. Let's check out the ingredients.

Thick beaten rice flakes, these have been dipped in buttermilk for 15-20 minutes in curd and sieved.

Grated carrots, green peas, grated white pumpkin, sugar and salt to taste.

And for the tempering, we need asafetida, sesame seeds, and mustard seeds.

Apart from that, we would require ginger garlic paste and green chili paste.

It's a very simple recipe.

Take the beaten rice which has been soaked in buttermilk. Now add in a little sugar and grated white pumpkin. Mix it properly.

Next, add in green peas and carrots.

Add in salt to taste. You must make sure that you add in all the ingredients and then add salt.

In the meantime, we will prepare the tempering.

For tempering, you need a little oil.

The tempering is ready.

Put in mustard and sesame seeds, and a pinch of asafetida.

Let it stand for a moment, and then add the tempering on the mixture we created earlier.

Add red chili powder to taste and little turmeric to the mixture.

Turmeric will change color and give its unique taste as well. Mix well.

Once the mixture is ready, you can prepare the 'Handwa' (pancake).

For this, let's put some oil in a pan or on a griddle.

Now we will make 'Handwa' that is around 10 mm thick and 7 to 8 inches in diameter.

This is made just like we make the 'Uttapam' and 'Thalipeeth'.

Now you will cover it.

You have to cook it on both sides for 15-20 minutes.

The Handwa will turn golden and fluffy.

Now we have to serve it. We can serve the 'Poha Handwa' with curd.

Orange Eucalyptus Bath Salts

When making your own bath salts and scrubs, we recommend using only dead sea salts or Epsom salts. Dead Sea Salts contain a considerably smaller proportion of sodium chloride than other salts. Sodium chloride, which makes up 80% of regular sea salts, and most of the solar salt, kosher salt, and rock salt, do not offer therapeutic benefits and can also be harmful to people with high blood pressure and edema.

On the other hand, the balance of magnesium, potassium and calcium chlorides, and a comparatively high concentration of bromides in Dead Sea Salts are what make them beneficial. And recent studies show that bromides are a healing factor for psoriasis.

Epsom salts are also made up of magnesium sulfate. This ingredient is what pulls soreness from muscles, making them great for combating stress and relieving muscle aches. The magnesium also aids in the removal of acids through the skin. Now, here's a recipe so you can make your own!

Orange-Eucalyptus Bath Salts

Winter colds don't leave you with much to be desired. Lift your spirits, ease muscle aches, and help clear nasal passages with this bath salt blend.

Ingredients:

1 Cup Fine Sea Salt

1/2 tsp Liquid Vegetable Glycerin

1/2 Cup Epsom Salts

8 drops eucalyptus essential oil

8 drops sweet orange essential oil

Instructions:

Combine all the ingredients in a bowl and mix well. To use, simply add 4 to 6 Tablespoons of salts to a hot tub. Keep unused salts sealed in an airtight container.

3 Homemade Relaxing Herbal Bath Salt Recipes

As mothers, we spend almost all of our waking hours taking care of the children, cleaning the home, preparing meals and doing the family errands. When was the last time that you did something relaxing just for yourself? If you had to pause for a moment to think about your answer, then it has been too long.

When I take time out just for myself, I enjoy taking a long hot bath. I like to fill up my bathtub with some homemade bath salts and while I am soaking, read a good book. These baths help to relax me after a long busy day.

The following recipes are really easy to make.

Relaxing Lavender

2 cups Epsom Salts

1/2 cup sea salts

1/4 cup baking soda

4 drops of Lavender Essential Oil

Mix Epsom salts, baking soda and sea salt together in a large bowl. Stir in the Lavender Essential Oil until salt mixture is coated. Let air dry and then pour into a container with a lid. Use a 1/4 to 1/2 cup of bath salts under warm running water.

Romantic Rose

2 cups Epsom Salts

1/2 cup sea salts

4 drops of red or pink soap coloring

4 drops of Rose Essential Oil

Mix together the first 2 ingredients in a large glass bowl. Stir in the soap coloring and essential oil until well blended. Use a 1/4 to 1/2 cup of the mixture under warm running water.

Hydro-Therapy Salts

2 cups Epsom Salts

1 cup sea salts

6-8 drops of blue soap coloring

Mix together the first 2 ingredients in a large glass bowl. Stir in the soap coloring until well blended. Use a 1/2 cup of the mixture under warm running water.

Himalayan Pink Sea Salt Recipes

Himalayan Pink Sea Salt can be cooked on, cooked in, served on and sprinkled over food or included in spice mixtures for just about any dish you can dream of! Recipes using Himalayan Sea Salt are becoming increasingly popular and therefore are beginning to gain in number, though there are literally thousands of recipes waiting to be discovered! It's solid, naturally compressed nature is due to concealment for eons, under extreme pressure, deep under the Himalayan mountains that allow for more various forms and uses of the salt that can be found in most other salts. Certain forms of this special salt can be used for a unique, gourmet presentation of your food while adding varying degrees of rich, salty flavor to any dish.

One such form is the Himalayan Pink Salt Grill, Block or Kitchen Slab. Salt grills provide a unique, gourmet cooking experience, as you actually grill your food right on a natural salt block! The saltiness the food acquires using this technique can be adjusted with the use of varying amounts of liquids, such as oils or juices, and also depends on the amount of moisture inherent to the type of food you are cooking. This last factor is best explained by taking into consideration the liquid content of fruit vs. the liquid content of a dryer food such as a London Broil steak. Put simply, the more moisture you place on a salt slab, tray or grill, with your food, the more salt will be absorbed and the saltier your food will taste.

Himalayan Salt bowls can be used as a dish in which to toss salads, adding a touch of salty flavor to fresh greens or even fresh fruit salads. They can also be used to serve cold soups and even ice cream, for a sweet, salty treat with an exceptionally mouthwatering presentation your guests and family will love. Salt bowls and plates, along with blocks and slabs, can also be used to salt cure foods. There are even Sushi presentation blocks to chill, cure and/or serve your signature Sushi dishes on.

Both fine and coarse grain Himalayan Pink Sea Salt can, of course, be used to season any dish you like and add a special touch to beverages such as Margaritas and other salty drinks. This granular form of the salt can be used to make salt brines for fish and can also be mixed with other ingredients for salt-crusted dishes, such as whole fish cooked in sea salt. It can be smoked, for added flavor, and even dissolved in water for use as the ever popular Sole Therapy Drink.

Basic Bath Salt: This is the simplest way of making a bath salt. In this recipe, instead of a cup of fine good pool rock salt, you can put a cup Epsom salt. Additionally, you can put some scents to your liking such as lime, apple, coconut, Ylang Ylang oil. The alternative is countless.

- Ingredients:

1 cup sea salt

1 cup pool rock salt

2 cup Baking Soda

2. Relaxing Bath Salt: After a stressful day, it is the right time to relax and chill out. Lavender and sage will ease out all your worry and tenseness!

- Ingredients:

1 cup Epsom salt

1 cup Dead sea salt

2 cup Baking Soda

10 drops Lavender oil

5 drops Coconut oil

10 drops Clary sage oil

3. Romantic Bath Salt: Here comes the great idea for a sweet Valentine!

- Ingredients:

1 cup Epsom salt

1 cup Dead sea salt

2 cups baking soda

20 drops rose essential oil

10 drops Lavender essential oil

4. Pain Relieving Bath Salt: When you have aches or pain somewhere on your body, just take a bath as followed, peppermint, eucalyptus will ease your pain and raise your spirit.

- Ingredients:

1 cup Epsom salt

1 cup Dead salt

20 drops Peppermint essential oil

10 drops Eucalyptus essential oil

10 drops Lavender oil

- Here's how:

In a small bowl, place all the salts together, add the soda and drop the oils. Keep mixing till all the ingredients evenly distributed. Store in a well-sealed container to keep out moisture.

Salt Water Swimming Pool

Are you pondering buying a new swimming pool in the upcoming summer? Or perhaps your just wishing to convert that old pool to a newer salt water pool? In today's day and age, most people are talking about going green, and by converting or buying a salt-water pool, your helping the environment and saving yourself money in the long run. With a salt water pool, all you do is simply add your salt directly to the water, from there the water will pass through a generator and through a process it then splits up into sodium and chlorine which is what a pool needs to stay clean.

 Most people with allergies or skin problems to chlorine, have switched to a salt water swimming pool because it seems to be less of a problem than adding all the other chemicals as well as chlorine. Not only does a salt-water pool help them with their allergies, it also takes less work to keep them up and running than regular pools. The cost of salt is also considerably less than your average pool.

Do Salt Water Swimming Pools Work?

By nature, 'Salt' is Sodium Chloride. The method by which a salt-chlorine generator works is that it applies a process of electrolysis to the dissolved salt in the water as it passes through a pool's filter system. This electrolysis takes away the 'sodium' part of salt and what is left is chloride or chlorine. This form of chlorine is very natural and does not have the normal byproducts you will find with other types of chlorine- ie. red eyes, strong odor, etc.

WHAT ARE THE BENEFITS OF A SALT WATER SYSTEM?

What makes this system so enjoyable for pool-owners is that because the chlorine is produced and dispersed into the pool on such a consistent basis, it is much more difficult for the water to get cloudy or develop algae, and as we all know, algae will make or break just how much one enjoys swimming pool ownership. This consistency in the chlorine levels also makes pool maintenance much easier due to the fact that one does not need to check the chlorine levels on a daily basis, nor is adding of chlorine tablets or weekly "shocking" of the pool water necessary. I can personally attest to these benefits considering my ownership of a composite (fiberglass) pool in my yard with a salt-chlorine generator. In fact, I did not have to add any chlorine or shock this past summer, despite the fact that our pool had up to 19 children at one time and was used every day by my two children as well as the rest of the neighbors. No one complained of red eyes and my water maintained excellent clarity throughout the whole season. Never was there a trace of algae. My pool is roughly 17,000 gallons and we only added two bags of salt the entire season. Our chemical cost for the entire year was less than $50! Needless to say, my wife thinks that salt chlorinators are the greatest thing since sliced bread and I would tend to agree.

ARE THERE ANY DRAWBACKS TO USING A SALT CHLORINATOR IN MY POOL?

Although there are very few drawbacks to salt-water chlorination, I'll list here what I've been able to observe. The initial investment one will spend on a good salt system will fall somewhere between $1000-$2500. Although this may sound like a lot, it really isn't when you figure that it will save on average over $500 a season for those using a different method in sanitation. The system will quickly pay for itself over just a few swimming seasons, but even if there weren't monetary benefits, it certainly is worth its weight in gold when one figures the time and stress that are alleviated with its implementation.

One other drawback with salt is that it does not work as well in a concrete/gunite pool. This is because studies have proven salt-chlorine to be five times more abrasive than regular chlorine on concrete surfaces. This means that a concrete pool owner will have to replaster their pool at a quicker rate if salt water is used. This principle does not apply to composite(fiberglass) pool owners though, with salt water having no negative impact on the longevity of the pool's structure.

DOES THE POOL WATER TASTE LIKE SALT?

Yes, the water does taste like salt, but the salinity levels are very low, and just slightly noticeable. I would certainly not consider the salt levels to be uncomfortable nor distracting.